The Dream Escape:

A Voice Of Awareness

David R McCovey

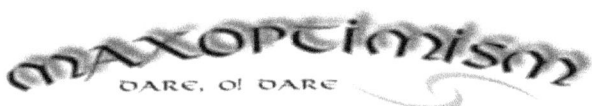

MAXOPTIMISM
DARE, O! DARE

Printed in the United States of America

The Dream Escape: A Voice of Awareness, 2nd Edition /
*1st Edition was independently published in September 2008;
+ISBN 9781440411007

David R McCovey, author
United States of America
www.amazon.com/author/maxotimism

David R McCovey's Books:

(Watch for Author's New Releases)

In Memory of:

Zeola

David R McCovey

Contents:

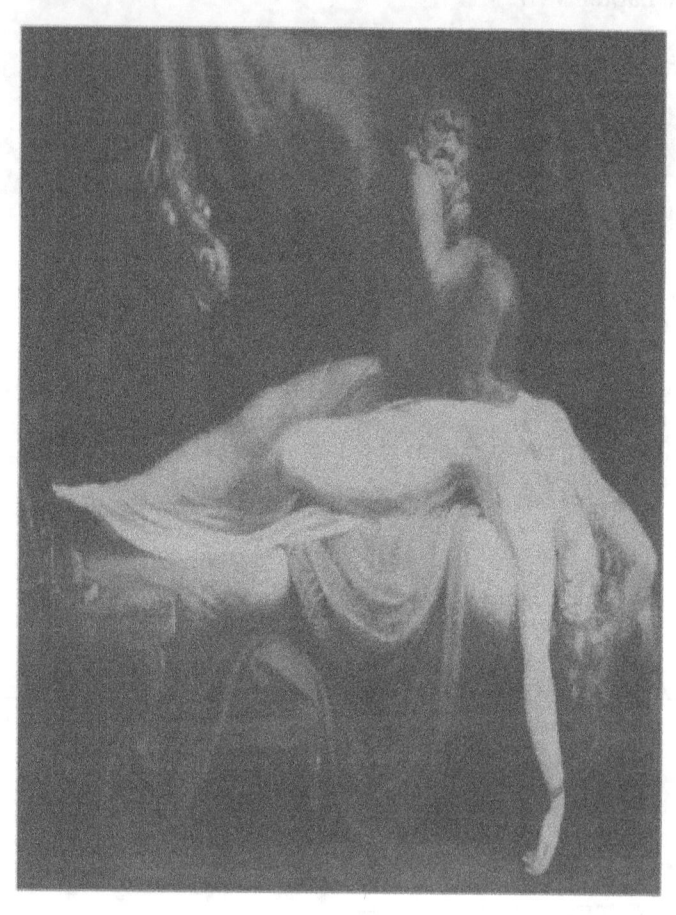

The Dream Escape:
A Voice of Awareness

"*Jung proposed two basic approaches to analyzing dream material: the objective and the subjective.*

In the objective approach, every person in the dream refers to the person they are: mother is mother, girlfriend is girlfriend, etc. In the subjective approach, every person in the dream represents as aspect of the dreamer.

Jung argued that the subjective approach is much more difficult for the dreamer to accept, but that in most good dream work, the dreamer will come to recognize that the dream characters can represent an unacknowledged aspect of the dreamer.

Thus, if the dreamer is being chased by a crazed killer, the dreamer may come eventually to recognize his own homicidal impulses.

Gestalt therapists extended the subjective approach, claiming that even the inanimate objects in a dream can represent aspects of the dreamer," Wikipedia.

The Dream Escape

Proem

To imagine that a great number of psyches have been stifled, or saved, depending on severity, or points-of-view, by phobia wouldn't be such a hair raising traipse down parlous slopes. Phobia, like the fear of snakes, for example, could be debilitating yes but also can warn of danger in them there tall grasses.

"In a predisposed person if there is no adaptation for conversion and still for the purpose of defense a separation of an unbearable idea from its affect is undertaken, the effect must then remain in the psychic sphere.

The weakened idea remains apart from all association in consciousness, but its freed affect attaches itself to other not in themselves unbearable ideas, which on account of this 'false' connection become obsessions.

This is in brief the psychological theory of the obsessions and phobias," Sigmund Freud, Austrian Neurologist [1856 - 1939].

Joseph Jules DeJerine, French Neurologist [1849 - 1917], accords phobias in psychoneurotics occur as a result of the misinterpretation of various unpleasant or distressing sensations or experiences. He view, for example, food phobias may occur as a result of attaching an erroneous significance to distressing sensations about the stomach, such as a feeling of pressure or heaviness.

As highlighted phobia causation has scores of viewpoints yet one thing is of common,– complex phobias, as social phobia, are more likely to cause anxiety. By inference phobia is an anxiety disorder.

In relation morbid fear, by assumption, in severe afflicted mind can trigger maladaptive delusionary fantasies, or grandiose vivid dreams, or even lurid daymares in association with 'fight or flight' stimuli contradictory to what lie in reality, an experience involving the perception of something not present.

Ascension of vivid dreams application to elude morbid fear, conscious contends, exemplify the psyche adaptability, its fluidity, in its quest to remain sane, or, to a larger degree, in its unwillingness to confront phobia. The price paid? –Anxiety in the awaken state.

If fear of flying, for example, keeps a soul grounded then there would be no need to be concerned about plane crashes, logically speaking, but that phenomenon, that phobia, can torpefy when air travel is been highlighted during the holiday season.

If that fear becomes severely morbid social avoidance may follow, the mind can then seek to remain vibrant in sphere of maladaptive delusionary fantasy, or grandiose vivid dreams, which by argument can be triggered by a simple phone call.

A bigger concern however is– residual impressions left upon receptive brain by assiduous adaptation could soon be firmly maintained despite contradicting reality with the resulting idiosyncrasy been delusion.

"Vivid dreams can mean there's a lot of deep emotional work and healing going on, and can leave us feeling more tired in the morning. More

dreaming means more REM sleep which can mean less deep sleep." Dr
Nerina Ramlakhan, physiologist and sleep therapist.

Then, results of 'less deep sleep' could however be the
causation, the noxious, of distorted thinking such as false beliefs in
social interactions— i.e. feelings of been judged. Signs of social
phobia.

It is estimated that some 15 million, nationally, adults suffer
extreme anxiety— phobia, in social interactions so severe they become
repressed by fear. And, the lack of deep sleep may provoke symptoms in vulnerables.

Distress over social interactions, for example: public speaking, in extremes may provoke the loosening of associations possible
morphing into dreams that is, by nature, delusionary, or psychotic, in
effort to dissociate, mental dissociation, from fear. During which
there is a complete lack of insight into susceptible true state of conscious reality.

Viable connections have been tracked between anxiety
disorders— phobia, and changes in sleep, lack of deep sleep, cycles.
Phobia may cause disturbing dreams and induce higher likelihood of
sleep disruptions.

Loss of self-reflective capacity, a causation of phobia, may
indeed become provocateur of lucid dreams, if severe. Severity of
phobic fears can indeed provoke hallucinations. Triggered by a
simple telephone call.

*"Anxiety dreams are more than just anxiety related. Our dreams
are a way for us to process information from the day, the week, the month,*

the years. They are also a way to process thoughts and feelings that are front of mind by attaching them to stories," Joshua Klapow, PhD, Clinical Psychologist.

In extremes, attaching thoughts and feelings to stories can apply equally to feelings of fear related to phobia as causation of dreams turning hallucinatory in nature.

Devising of alter-ego, for example, psyche moored to delusion becomes heroic in anxiety related dreams as rebuttal against phobic stimulus. Here again thoughts can be seen as lacking insight into susceptible true state of consciousness.

It deserves repeating:—

"Loss of self-reflective capacity, a causation of phobia, may indeed become provocateur of lucid dreams, if severe. Severity of phobic fears can indeed provoke hallucinations. Triggered by a simple telephone call."

David R McCovey

I

"When considering the circuitry of a brain and, in tune, human psychology, accord studies, some of the chemicals —noradrenalin— that contribute to the 'fight or flight' response may indeed also be present in varying positive emotional states as: happiness and excitement. It then makes sense that the elevated arousal state experienced during a state of exhilaration may also be experienced in a state of fear; — terror!"

Terror Is Close...

A void in darkness is terrifying. It hadn't been such an unusual day, atypical he would say, up and until the triggering phone call came. That damn phone call, that suffocating phone call, hit like a ton.

He was readying himself for a stress free evening having the house to himself for the first time ever; despite the weather.

It carry winds beyond 55 miles per hour, tornado patterned swirls uprooted swaying trees, and slung shingles off rooftops. The not so un-rare spring thunderstorm's bountiful clouds portly with rain came ashore from off the ocean waters of the southern shores.

Its howling raging winds, echoing thunderous booms, and pounding raindrops dreary this usually vibrant home at a time he — Thomas, was phobic immobilized.

Some aversions can be debilitating, devitalizing, more so in the guise of grim darkness as it was for him this bewitching night... horrifying.

Specially in an empty home that is normally rocked by pitter-patter of little feet hurrying about, shouting voices in roughhouse play, and too a doting wife's sweet aura. Now silence plaster these unfussy beige walls.

Gripped by it — anxiety, sleep remaining at bay, panicky shivers spur sweat socked bedding, aversion fed terror overwhelm this somber night before one of the most sacred days of lore form of persuasion, although not entirely faith filled, the coming of morning too, as it is, brings the celebrating of the resurrection.

But this night, this night of trepidation, however terror encroach out direful darkness bedaubing psyche conscious gloom, and it, terror, approaches from the void as agitated brain floods nerve cells with 'fight or flight' hormones.

Though some 86 billion neurons in a brain are connected to each other, and each has approximately

10,000 inputs connection, and through this circuit electrical activity flows from one cell to the next, to the next, as it is, for him, now happening. Intense dread can foster non-response to a anxiety rich brain's output connection, or warning signals.

"Run!" shouts came from quickening sinking mind.

Try, try, try as muscling mind did the body, flaccid, couldn't or wouldn't respond to adrenaline stimuli approaching terror aroused. The psyche, always prone for self-preservation, attempts its escape into sphere beyond sub-conscious.

For years doting wife of 28 years had strived to get him more involved with their parish but he was always to busy, to tried, to something to involve himself with additional affairs, — not been so devoted.

So it was foreboding, ominous, to hear his own dubious voice — "Do you forsake me?" question, spoken in prayerful strain. "It's more than I can bear," wheezed out shadowed breath.

Pounding heart raced, thrumming in reverberating ears, the exact moment an explosion of thunder, powerfully loud, shook windowpane in the 'double hung' window looking out.

Next to plush Ames wood framed bed — king size, a Ames 3 drawer Louis XIV nightstand held a tall tumbler halved with ice chilled water that had rippled due the magnitude, the rumbling.

All the vast night gobbling sky was soon after lit by electrifying streaks of illuminating lightning.

Throughout the greater city sirens could be heard blaring here-to-there when the last targeting streak touched ground striking a distribution transformer causing citywide blackouts, intensifying the dense blackness phobia is now entombed.

Amplifying the dreadful void encroaching out the subliminal darkness.

Cold sweat ran the length of steely cheeks, he could not wipe at it, could not move, and was indifferent to the weather ravaging the stormy outside that could not transfix consciousness.

Terror was reaching out the void, reaching out skeletal claws, reaching for him.

"No! Go away," ringing ears was sure they heard willful voice cry, was sure, frightful mind think, it heard willful voice scream, scream that had no actual sound though rich in mental volume.

The air in Bohemian fashioned bedroom turns musty & stuffy, smell of rotten flesh that lacerated nasal sense of smell hallucinating sanity was sure seeps from ground storied home foundation stands, suffocating nostril inapt breaths.

"I can't breathe," was heard proclaimed in divorced throbbing head; he was sure.

The constant rain had lessened, the whipsawing winds now blew mildly, still thunder rumble in grumpy skies of fretful night with resounding echoes, this last one seems to pierce forehead's prickling skull.

Dazzling lightning that follows stentorian blast sprays white flashes back dry twitching eyes just before knockout came, —he lies unconscious.

II

"The two important constituents of dreams are the sequence of perceptions and the presence of hallucinatory imagery."

Illusive Wings...

Clouds rangy gauzy. Brilliant ball of eclipsing fire high noonday picturesque, gentle azure, ineffable sky, cast fierce sunrays down on basking beachgoers, onto reflective turquoise waters of the western shores, along golden coast at Cambrian Bay — bright & blinding to naked eyes.

White sand hot grains ooze through wrinkled toes with each gangling step.

In solace with noonday sunshine enthralled ears listen to summer's lively symphony — splash of rippling waves coming ashore, chattering voices of tanning sunbathers lazy improvisation, screaming kee-eeeee-arr of a soaring red-tailed hawk probing Cambrian canyon, barking growls of eared seals basking on distant sea rocks, too nature's lyrical whiff of ocean breeze.

All these polyphonic sounds, these pleasurable sounds, pleases absorbing senses save the sense of spellbound touch, his was spellbound, attentive only to those arresting fingers interlaced with his longing stubbies.

Too, the musical sound of her name exhaled from avid lips was sweet & salty, taste of caramel candies.

Her spirit, the thought of her, gave life to slowing steps, — returns the hands of time back to period of reckless youth. She has always been the one love although work and other obligations kelp them apart for stretches, sometimes years.

It had been more than six months since their last tryst he remember it as it was yesterday; — Rome.

In the ancient land they had spent two weeks battling crowds as they too wondered from one tourist site to another, to another like the Renaissance Palaces, and ancient ruins as the Ruins of Paestum.

They visited the Vatican's Plus-Clementine Museum and stared in awe at the Statue of La Coon then dined at Les Eloiles, known as 'a garden in the sky', where they feasted on Mediterranean cuisine.

And in their Roman Palazzo, its lobby decorated with murano chandeliers, columns and marble busts, made love in early dawn at the St Regis Grand.

Beneath the night skies of Italy they savored cocktails and live music while gliding on the Tiber River cruising past ancient sites as Castel Sant'Angelo and St Peter's Basilica.

She would snuggle against him, in his embrace, and the lights of the city would glimmer in concert with adoring moonlight— all was right under venerating stars that offered, as she, dazzling entice.

By the end of their interlude his regards, his affection, his love for her was affirming. Although he knew the claims of their profession was restrictive, limiting, to his aspiration.

Now, wanting to savor this moment, this time, to nestle in it, desiring mind was winging distant terrains and barely heard the faint tenor of her baiting voice, though he adore its sound, when she spoke of her latest travels.

They both had reserved this time, marked it on their calendars, and settled on Cambrian when she had telephoned saying she needed to see him.

He had taken the reins, had made the plans, and was now grasping her silken hand thinking if there was but one, one person, designed for each created human, to be that one and only mate, he was certain that she was conceived for the purpose, like gloves for hands, of his comfort.

"I have a surprise for you," he voices mischievously playful.

"What kind of surprise?" she inquires urgently.

"You'll have to wait. We have reservations a Gaetano for seven I will pick you up at six-thirty make sure you are ready I wouldn't want to have the wait; not long without doubt," again playfully conveyed.

"It'll be worth the wait," she counters.

"I'm sure, but let's try to make the reservation time."

After awhile, they had been pensively lying on the sand, beach towel beneath them, her head resting on his bare chest. He reposition to sit with legs crossed and folded at the knees, she leans against him enjoying the picture perfect view of the waters of the western shores, the mountains terrain enveloping coastal contours, and too the uninhibited antics of pelicans hilarious play before turning to face him, to look into his smiling eyes.

Together, in concert, they became oblivious, unconcern, of any other body as their conversation deepens the world seems to become uninhabited.

He was in an absolute, total, state of bliss hypnotized by her, by those reflective light brown eyes reflecting flaring sunlight.

For some unexplained reason, he couldn't say why, an omen brushes him, it felt as though he was in the crosshairs of an unseen, unforgiving, sniper waiting for a clear kill shot.

Taking notice of the faraway, bizarre, look that had seized his grayish eyes, the worry wrinkles deforming his forehead, and the tension marking his once endearing embrace, she held his hardy face in sensual hands, kisses him flirtatiously, slowly, softly, on full lips drawing him back to her.

He had no defense, no resistance, no hostility to her conspiring obsession, racing searching fingers around outline of nudging breasts, stopping to pinch jutted nipple sending tantalizing shockwaves.

Low soiled moans escapes busying lips when open to allow for probing tongue's incursion.

The bandeau bikini top no longer held a breast, it had been replaced by a jealous hand that covers its exposure, she was not opposed to exhibitionism, indecent exposure, this make-out's euphoric feelings could have led to, wanting to lead to, if he hadn't swiftly stop, ropes his mannish arms around her kinetic waist lifting her as he stood.

Again that ominous omen stiffen him, alarms primitive instincts, and liken to a grazing prey in perilous wilderness cranes vigilant neck to search amidst mingling sheep for that skulking predator lurking in the bush.

Seeing none his attention was drawn, enticed, she had bowed over, back to her, she was gathering their things, the way light of the shifting sun flared her melanin rich skin, it radiates, he wanted to capture, time stamp, halt earth's rotation, so that the image would be forever immortalized.

He pulls the Nikon FA camera, he would otherwise have been a photographer, choose what he considers as the best camera on the market, out its case and starts snapping like a photographer on a photo shoot whose subject was a world renowned model.

She plays along bring out, parading, her girlish, unashamed, un-bashful, spirit. With it she puts on display the reason why men, grown men, drool when that white bandeau bikini rides the right spot, high-lighting the sling of flowing reddish hair that teases wanton eyes— a tantalizing prize.

"Breathtaking," he mutters then froze having to have glance over to where they had parked, caught a glimpse of sunlight bouncing off the binoculars' lens.

Nerve ends became glutted, hair fibers on back of straining neck stood on ends, with adrenalin.

He had only gotten a glimpse before the guy drove away, he was certain nonetheless that the man had been watching, spying, on them, he would however remember that black BMW 3 Series, he got a good look at it, at its plates.

After his own Mercedes-Benz had been loaded he snaps one final photo of her sitting on the hood then drove to her hotel, the Clarion Hotel & Spa, near Old

Seafarer's Wharf resisting, fighting, the temptation to go to her suite.

Instead he drew her into his arms, held her close, inhales her fading perfume as she allows his audacious hands to explore her welcoming, her desiring, brash bosom.

"I'll have you later. Six-thirty reservations; be ready," he whispers before walking away leaving her standing in lobby watching him go through glass doors.

She lands back in her suite, after an elevator ride to the top floor, slips off the bikini, wraps herself in the hotel provided cotton fabric robe, picks up the telephone receiver and made the call.

David R McCovey

III

*"Darkness shines luminous light
upon... Blue Moon,
mimic voices howlin' in mist
of perpetual blindness at thy whispers"*

Unchecked Anxiety...

With the day still been fairly young he had parked blocks away from the hotel, on Lighthouse Boulevard, so they could walk and window shop the unique shops fronting the Clarion.

It was late day sunny, not as hot, a cooling breeze, blowing off the waters of the western shores, had come ashore which is normal as the day begins its decent and fog starts forming over the bay. He covers the distance in much less time than it took them to walk it. Nearing the spot, he took out the key, presses the remote button heard the click of the door lock — he slide into the driver seat pushes button to the sunroof as he drove away from the curve.

First stop was to be Gaetano to not only confirm the reservation but also too make additional arrangements, — a special bottle of her favorite wine was to be chilled; roses, deep red ones, was to be coordinated for delivery after the main course had been completed.

He met with Alberto Greco, a colorful character, manager of Gaetano who, in his deep Brooklyn accent, assured that everything would be arranged to his satisfaction. Even with Alberto's guarantee he still was left with feelings of uneasiness. This evening had to be perfect.

Minutes later, sitting in his Mercedes 300 CE outside the restaurant, he switches on the Alpine 7279 ms stereo system, Marvin Gaye's 'Trouble Man' came blaring through the Pioneer speakers he turns down the volume, dials numbers into the Motorola car phone for his friend Paul— one ring then answering machine.

"Out of touch," his thinking.

He did however leave message reminding Paul, his friend, and plausible business partner, to pick up the gift he had obtained for Cynthia's, Paul's wife, birthday, and too remind him that they would be arriving late, hours, to the celebration.

He pulls away from the curb, turns the volume up on the stereo Miles Davis' 'Autumn Leaves' now blare the speakers. It was but a short drive, half-hour, from the restaurant to his Surfside home where he had wanted her to stay while in town but she insisted on the Clarion.

Autumn Leaves was the perfect ambient sound,

it eased some of the tension, for the drive. The drive went east, along Dela Vina Way, he pulls to a stop at the intersection at Broadway — the light was red, where roving eyes spots, identifies, the car, the black car, the black BMW 3 Series, the same black BMW 3 Series he had seen at the beach, the black BMW 3 Series with the man that he was sure had been spying on them.

The driver of that black BMW 3 Series turns his head, his ash brown crew cut head, towards him held briefly his mocking stare, again the rush of adrenalin floods alerted nerve ends causing prickles to creep up knotting spine.

And when he — the man, gave a half smile half smirk it was enough of a confirmation, — "this guy is up to something, something no good," he — Thomas, muttered.

He, now fully alert, was on guard, observant of anything, any person, that looks suspicious, out the ordinary, or out of place.

The light turns green he was on his way with the guy's face stuck on his mind it was something about this stranger something familiar all his experienced facilities points to something dangerous.

He made a left turn onto Lowell, a residential street, his home was about midway of the next block on Hilliard, so engrossed in thought he almost missed the turn to his driveway, then when the strain of anxiety confiscated resolve he made a u-turn in middle of the road causing a oncoming car to slam its brakes and too veer, to miss hitting him.

She was all he could think of, to get to her, to ensure her safety. The guy had been spying on them what if it was her he was after what if he has already gotten to her.

While anxiety drunken nerve ends continued to be swamped with stress hormones his lead foot laid on the accelerator.

Nested on rugged coastline, Cambrian, this one-time center of the sardine packing industry, now a tourist coastal resort, and naturalist retreat, host the quality of life normally associated with artists, novelists, and poets, yet still famous for outdoor adventures rich with sea and land organisms, has on average very little major crime.

The police department here is small in comparison to larger cities, so when he, travelling at speeds in excess of 70 mph in 35 mph posted zones, saw those flashing red lights' blaring siren speeding towards him in his rearview mirror he thought about not stopping then quickly rejected the foolish temptation.

Before he could come to a complete stop, however, another patrol car cuts in front of him from a side street, he slams on the brakes so as to not slam into the cruiser.

"Damn," cursing, his mind racing, feelings of

impending doom, not his but hers, swept over leaving behind restive fragments. He was self-assumed.

Persons, milling, stopped to gawk then was hurried about, as motorist was detoured.

Late-day sun had moved lower in fuzzy evening sky, while shadows, elongated, made suspenseful the coming dusk; the settling gloom. A wayward crow lands on over-hanging limb of a holly tree, he noticed it, it squawked then flew away.

Oceanic aromatics, salty sulphury, gust through sheared hedges, fan palms, downed windows, and opened sunroof on his cream 300 CE coupe.

His mind raced.

That mocking smirk, that menacing smile, on the stranger's brawny face burn itself in his teetering thoughts, his galloping thoughts, thoughts that was also wondering— "How was he going to explain his reason for speeding?" "Was the mere fact that he harbor suspicion about some stranger, a stranger he had not before laid eyes, intent enough a reason so as to not be ticketed?" His mind raced.

Anxiety churns vexing innards.

IV

"ideally consideration would be amplified, not anesthetized, in humanity."

The Lost of Control...

Aggression drips the officer who had cut in front of him, the one whom he nearly slammed into, had drawn his pistol and taken cover behind his cruiser.

He— Thomas, notice also the officers, now numbering four patrol cars, at his rear was also aiming their weapons in his direction and, although it was not yet dark, he was besieged by the brilliance of spotlights.

Scattered mind was trying to find reasoning, justification, for their militant actions when the commanding shouts grudges appalled senses— "Turn off the engine. Take the keys, throw them out the window. Then put both hands on the steering wheel.

Do it NOW!" — the commands came from a throaty voice at his rear.

Taken aback, shocked, by this display of aggressiveness, this hostility, due the fact that he had weapons aiming at him, the commands didn't at first register in construing brain; he was slow to respond.

"DO IT NOW!" he heard a now frantic voice call out.

After tossing the keys his hands gripped the steering wheel tightly, white knuckle tight, as another command, "Keep your eyes straight ahead," came from the same frantic voice, — it had moved to the passenger side of the car.

Suddenly the passenger door swing open at the same instant he felt cold steel, barrel of a .38 pistol, on the side of his cringing neck.

"Get Out!" the throaty voice behind the barrel commands.

Anxiety turns towards resentment, resentment to indignation by this uncalled for treatment he views as unreasonably over-the-top for a simple traffic viola-tion. Even the god-awful screams of the sirens was becoming nauseating.

"On the ground," came another command.

He shrugs then got down. While lying prone on hot hard concrete he felt a knee press down onto the small of his flatten back, felt handcuffs cuff his sweat dampened wrists together, and himself lifted to befuddled feet.

He was then shoved, forcefully pushed, in direction of a waiting patrol car with, he suspected, a plain clothed policeman driving, was then ordered to get in.

He was sped away.

In matters of minutes he found himself stopped for speeding on narrow neighborhood roads to now setting handcuffed in back of a patrol car for reasons he could not find. It didn't take long however for the suddenness of the police actions to fade, and for nagging questions to again invade addled psyche.

No one had bother to read him his rights, nor ask for identification, drivers' license was at the ready, truth is no one had spoken to him outside the few commends hurled at him.

Perplexed, mystified, racing mind unable to find justification lapsed into wild guessing.

"Are you taking me into custody?" "Why?" "What's the charge?" "Shouldn't someone have spoken to me before placing me under arrest?" he barked a series of questions at the officer. No response came.

"Yes I admit to speeding, but why the warlike treatment?" his question again went unanswered.

Burning eyes stares at the back of the officer, who seem to have been oblivious of his presence, reddish curls filled head hoping for acknowledgement, for answers. But the officer was steadfast, his attention transfixed ahead, on his driving – maybe.

"Please officer; I can explain, I was responding to an emergency is the reason for my speeding. I have a friend at the Clarion Hotel that is in danger. I need to go there to check on her, to ensure she is safe," he pleads calmly, still the officer gave no indication, no hint, that he was even aware of his existences.

He leans back, his back firmly against the seat as the cruiser winds its way along the city streets, peering out onto the passing landscape. His mind racing.

"Officer!" again he tries to get some kind of response.

Perception lapse unto the plexus of uneasiness, the darkness of misgivings. Apprehension, boiling in dimple of gurgling gut, paved the berm to foreboding hinterlands where recklessness repudiates wisdom's mindful vigil.

He lays onto his side, manage to get his feet onto the seat, then starts kicking at the right side door; at the window.

Pissed, a-washed in animus, these actions had no obvious effect except on the handcuffs, they seems to have tighten cutting deeper into his throbbing wrist, his inflamed hands had gone numb no feelings was left in his fingers.

And liken to a trapped beast caught in hunter's

snare, his mind plunges into the bowels of the untold.

The creep of panic seized reins of his descending thoughts, his totality, when feeling the smoothness beneath the traveling tires change, the officers had turned onto a wooden pier, with the separation between cedar planks making for a bumpy ride.

Bump... bump... bump..., they traveled length of the weathered two lane pier in nondescript area tenanted by fish processing fisheries, and warehousing, where crews on fishing boats offload their bountiful catch. The air was thick of fishy tang. Seabirds, seems in the hundreds, linger in wait to grab a tasty treat.

"Hey!" "Hey man! where the fuck are you taking me?"

The cruiser moved slowly, tacitly, along its track coming to a stop near the very end, it was a fenced off area the posted sign read: "Restricted Area Keep Out".

The gates was swung open by a sentry dressed in navy blue coveralls tucked into a pair of Bates black leather boots, they passed through without fanfare, nor words. They drove the additional stretch in seconds coming to stop front of an old tin building, the officer switched off the engine, poised, snapping his head and neck from side-to-side in an apparent attempt to release tension, got out walks around to back opens the trunk.

The handcuffs was really biting into his wrist, making ever effort to get blood to his hand, which lacks feeling, he switch positions leaning forward resting his head on the caging. The trunk slammed shut, his head was raised by the sound and impact.

The officer stood at the rear momentarily then came around to the right side opens the rear door reaches in grabbed hand full of shirt at the collar pulls him practically out of the vehicle.

It was soon after his noise and mouth was covered with a cloth, a damp cloth, that everything went completely, instantly, black.

David R McCovey

V

"Hence to vigorously cogitate myriad, opposite,
of matters lent evolution of said unknowns
nil circumspection, foresight, for certainty innumerable"

Weakness Unseen...

It was the pounding, the pounding throb of a damn migraine topped with queasiness quarreling with a queer stomach, plus the wane of chloroform affect, that cause lucidity to began to regain consciousness.

The mouth was dry, cloud fogged the brain, bowels hard to maintain, and eyes cloaked in darkness although psyche was semi-awake, semi-lucid.

"He's awake."

Through lingering dense fog, and groggy, at best, equilibrium, it penetrated fuzzy, disoriented, lucidity enough for recognition to grab hold so that the far-off sound of that recognized voice cleared the persisting ill-effect of chloroform intoxication.

The tightly fitted blindfold prevented sight from seeing her, but the mind knew, it had heard that voice on many occasions, could remember the very first time ears heard that sweet contralto tone.

It was some twenty years ago, they were both recruits, it was months after they had completed their post-graduate studies — he at Silverstone Postgraduate School in Cambrian Bay, and she upon receiving a doctoral degree from the University of Aurora in Gaines.

Both had been invited to come to Lang for a tour, and to meet identified persons, at the Conglomerate. It was during this two day period that they was introduced, and it was during that first meeting ears first heard the voice of the person that would come to mean so much.

Together, and individually, they have traveled the world, have survived danger in hostile countries, have extracted sensitive documents while under deep cover, also have arranged the assassination of murderous warlords, and have facilitated corruption among foreign government officials.

It was just hours ago that cherish clung to her every word, no doubt of mind who that raspy voice belonged, who's raspy contralto voice that had broken through the fog clouding total consciousness, the same voice belonged the person desire had made love to in the open night air of Rome beneath glittering stars...

Gloria!

Now curiosity had been befuddled, perplexed, clawing for insight.

"Who's there?" perplexity, in its anger, shouts out at the persons it knows was there.

"Take off the blindfold," her voice, her familiar voice, commands.

The mind races, dumb stricken, — "why is she here?" "is it possible she has a hand in this?" "where am I?" "is this some kind of sick joke?" bombarded by questions the laboring confused mind sort clarity, clarity that would ease rearing anxiety.

Suddenly the blindfold was lifted and removed the eyes struggle to focus, the hands, still cuffed, was chained to an eyebolt attached to a 4 x 8 attached to the wall.

"How's your head?" her voice came from distance, from across the room.

The eyes searches for her finding her at seat, at seat on what appears as a bale of netting, fish netting, at the same time, the same realism when senses noticed, paid attention to, the motion, the buoyancy of boating, and experience says they were on the high waters.

The mind, now clear, begins to access, to make notes, noting that it, and they, was on a boat, a fishing boat by the looks of it.

"What's going on here, Gloria?" "What are you doing here?" "Why am I here?" curiosity aims series of needling questions in her direction.

She respond by coming closer, close enough for curiosity to be distracted by her bulging breast, thirty-six voluptuous, filling a white button-down blouse — the two top buttons was undone, tucked into a pair of skin tight jeans that left no doubt about her curvy form, her fitness. She also wore a black vest that bulge on the left side. "Packing heat," experience knowing thoughts.

"Gloria what's happening here?" tone of demanding voice was strained.

This was the first time sight had seen her since leaving her at the Clarion, sanity had so been concerned, so worried, about her safety.

"Remove the restraint," she gesture to a man standing in the shadows who moves into light, unlocks, removes, the handcuffs that was still cutting circulation to thankful hands, few minutes later feelings returns, numbness had waned, and hands felt anew.

She walks towards him with eyes ablaze, smiling, stopping with only inches of separation then brushed teasing lips across uncertain, questioning, lips.

"I'm sorry it had to be done in such a fashion, but time is not on our side I had plans to bring you in at dinner the situation is changing as we speak," she offers a crude explanation.

"Bring me in on what?" tension that had muscles in rigid neck, clenched in anger, fighting waves of anxiety, eases. Sight searches for possible hidden messages in her gentle eyes, in her assured demeanor.

"Shortly we will rendezvousing at sea, from there a helicopter will fly us to Elsa Air Base where you will receive your brief," she reveals.

"At sea," thoughts intones, its suspicious been confirmed; they were indeed at sail.

"Bring me in on what?" curiosity quiz, tension eased, anxious neck muscles relaxes still nausea engulfs nostalgia feelings. Mind's memories of their recent time, just hours aged, together —"was it not real?"— tries, awry, to mesh then with what is now happening.

"Those things that was said was they not truthful?" "Had she been deceptive?" uncertainty inundates racing thoughts.

Shallow legs took a few steps backward, space was needed, her standing so close was confusing, throwing poise off balance, to already shaky reliance. It was troubling, distressing, that she would have a hand in its, as logic sees it, maltreatment.

Allegiance couldn't perceive itself condoning, allowing for, harm of her. She the passion of wanton awaken hours, and the luscious thing in sleep dreams that kelp nightmares at bay.

They had spent most of the day walking, or

lying on, the sandy beach of Cambrian Bay in all that time he didn't read in her voice, nor in her body language, a problem, a storm, was over the horizon. Has she gotten that good, that masterful, at manipulation, at masking intent? Or, as wit suspects, liken for Samson has she become his Delilah?

Hope didn't want to believe what they had, what they confess to having, was not real, anything to the contrary was unbalancing. Questions needs answers; answers needs to be assuring.

Due their shared history conjecture had convinced itself that the heart well knew her, knew her likes her dislikes, knew when she hid truth, knew the flavor of her lusting heart. Did she not just this very day snuggle against affection, show fondness care, and make noonday warmth magical? Was it not this same woman that now stands before revere with mystery winging untold tells?

For the first time, the very first time, since psyche had recognize her raspy contralto voice speak through the blindfold, and her decisive command to the guy standing in shadow, sight looks about, search, with trained eyes, the area in which it stood.

At first glance it appears to be an ordinary fishing vessel, they stood in the belly below deck this area would hold the catch-of-the-day if this boat was actually meant for catching fish, skepticism suspect not, it suspect that this boat, the boat that takes it out to sea, was outfitted and then lunched for clandestine activities although by law the Conglomerate was barred from operating within the boundaries of the United States, used mainly for interrogations.

Intellect couldn't get a fix on the number of persons topside. Gloria, the stoic guy who had removed the handcuffs, and to its surprise, its horror, sitting quietly, ominously, was the driver of that black BMW, and when probing eyes again gazed one-to-one senses was then again gasp by baleful omen, was the other body in this space.

Carlos is his name.

VI

"Into the glam— flumped as nonplus lamp life had succumb fore sat upon by likeable funk an' gorged by nubile solstice luminous kicks flicking vision-sweet crump— alluress effusing orbit dispelling gulping' slump I was convulsing love's smothering stomps gazing exquisite slumber in hump of dawn now thence laid brazen-faced in nimble arms— howls plume life's turn"

Veil Of Secrecy...

At a little over six feet tall his athletic 185 pounds physique, molded by years of intense training, & demanding field work, was ideal for deep cover.

He, however, had to look up standing next to Carlos, who stood in the vicinity of six feet eight inches, and tips the scale at around 300 pounds, to see into the man's light brown eyes.

He had often been in the present of men like Carlos, dangerous men, and from experience knew his specialty and it was not something he would wish to be on the receiving end, nor wish upon those he dislike.

Carlos, he inferred, was an interrogator whose

main specialty was to extract real time information from unlucky high value targets that finds themselves at his mercy. Many surely have died.

By not been in the direct employment of the Conglomerate, exactly, instead contractors, persons of Carlos' teams has ever, will ever, face prosecution for violating the rights, the human rights, of any, or for violating international laws simple due these men, mostly men, are ghosts their paper trails leads unto a black hole with countless chambers with death as its guardian.

Knowledge of whereabouts at any given time is known only by a very small number of senior shot callers, in fact only the director himself is privy to the full scope of their identity.

Unalike other clandestine exertions whose funding can eventually be traced to budgets of the Army, or the Navy, or other Intelligent Agencies, funding for these activities however, which has no budgetary account, are often funded secretly as part of the Force Development Research Funds Allocation, or, mainly, by piracy, thievery, for example his last assignment was funded in part by the thief of funds generated through the illicit drug trade bound for southeast Asia he often imagine the look on faces when that ship's container had been opened by the cartel.

Carlos had placed a hand, a powerful hand, on

his shoulder the move caught him perplexed but what Carlos said, "I'm so glad to meet a man with your resume," left him stunned that he, Carlos, would have had excess to his files meant that he was more then first appearance, and didn't know what to say, what was expected, so he gave a nod acknowledgement.

Carlos, as he saw, is a brawny, intimidating, man who radiates danger, who injects fear, and a man who is adept in psychological warfare, and he — Thomas, so hope that there wouldn't come a time he and this man would become enemies engaged in fight.

"I saw you at the beach, you were watching us," he said just as Carlos, boastfully, extends a congratulatory handshake.

"Yes, I was trying to be as obvious as possible," came the reply.

"Why?"

Carlos explodes in booming, blustery, laughter exerting pressure to his challenge filled handshake causing him— Thomas, to look down, and as he did he noted the contrast, the contrast between the swarthy rich hand grapping his dusky tawny hand trying to match Carlos' strength, determine to show that he could handle his business, had no fear, and as virile as any man.

This display of manly brutishness between two seasoned men was soon, and promptly, muted by a seasoned woman's touch. She had been watching hoping their struggle for dominance wouldn't get out of hand, this shit, she decides, have to wait for later. A hand atop theirs was all it took to bring down the temperature.

"Carlos why don't you go and see if things are all set," she directs.

"Gloria what's going on here?" he — Thomas, inquires when they were alone.

"You'll get your brief at Elsa."

"No; I need, I deserve, to know what's going on."

"I'm under strict orders, you will have to wait."

"Am I to assume you didn't call out the blue, out of desire to spend time together, to be with me?"

"I don't want you to think that. Yes I called knowing about the situation but I wanted to see you."

"What situation?"

"Your brief is awaiting at Elsa."

Her kiss was hungry, melting, unpretentious, leaving no doubt of her feelings shown in the essence of her flitting body's response to his fondling, aroused, fingers' trace, grasp, of her ample, amiable, behind.

"Don't think for one minute that I don't care," she whispers assurances.

Alerting buzz came through the speakers followed by a voice announcement — "Surfs up."

"Time to go," she said while handing him the blindfold. "Put it on," she instructed.

He starts to protest then decides to comply knowing it wouldn't do any good to argue though him deciding was helped by the fact that Carlos was back at his side and had a hand firmly on his shoulder.

"Why the blindfold?" he finally wanted to know.

"As you may realize this boat, and the crew topside, has an important mission its existence is unknown and must remain so even you must be able to deny laying eyes on either," it was Carlos who responds.

He— Thomas, allows himself to be led, led up and onto the top deck, there he could hear chattering voices, people moving about, and the helicopter hovering above. He felt the cool breeze swirling, the fresh air, and listens to the sound of waves splashing in the mellow ocean, with pleasure took a moment to inhale.

Persons, one on each side, took hold of tensed arms— "Relax sir, a lift basket is to your front we will help you in, don't worry we got you," an unfamiliar voice spoke its accent was of the eastern European region.

After he was securely in the basket he felt himself quickly become airborne rising and swaying in strong gusty whipping breeze, back and forth, to and fro, he sways. The sound of the rotor blades coming closer, closer, and closer, then with a sudden jolt he came to a hard stop.

"How was that?" that familiar voice asks. He smiles knowingly, that she was onboard was pleasing.

"Not bad; let's do it again," was his josh reply.

She took hold his hand, helps him climb out the basket, the basket was then cut loose and allowed to fall into the ocean, she gave signal to the pilot the pitch of the blades was altered the helicopter tips forward then took to flight.

His last trip to Elsa Air Base was some eight or nine years ago he remembers fondly the open ranch lands along the coast, and had enjoyed hiking the surrounding hills, exploring in some of the numerous canyons the area is populated. He was there during one of the testing phase of the Stonewall III and had the chance to view the ICBM launch during comprehensive exercises as a visiting instructor for a operational readiness training program.

Now that it was fact that he was returning to Elsa he hope for a chance to walk that stretch along the Pacific, walk it with Gloria.

Ten minutes into the flight, the boat, Carlos, and his team, was far out of sight, she gave the ok for him to remove the blindfold. He discovers that the pilot was the only other person onboard with he and Gloria.

"I hope that's the last time I need blindfolding," expressing his dislike.

"It was necessary in this case, Carlos insisted," she explains.

"Who's pulling your strings in this?"

She allows the question go without answer instead she looks out onto the night, they was still flying over water, at the passing lights along the shoreline.

"I didn't cancel the reservation," he, breaking silence, shouts over the noise of the rotors.

"What was the surprise?" she, without telling that the reservation had indeed been cancelled and removed from Gaetano's books, asks with interest.

"I will save it for another time, a better time," he, feeling dismay, offers suspense laced response.

The landing zone was void of ground crew when they arrive, it was in the darkest hours, they were met, and greeted, by a single liaison who hustled them into a vehicle that drove and left them at silo LF-02.

There they were soon greeted, in his southern droll, by a Colonial Seagraves who hustled them into the silo's elevator that descended eight floors beneath surface to open to a long vacant corridor, there they was left standing as the Colonial took the elevator back to the surface.

"What was your role, if any, in the planning of my abduction?" he, still bothered she was at anyway involved, asks probing for answers.

Before she could offer up an response the door

at the far end swung open and a man, a frail looking man wearing thick glasses and disarming smile, came marching towards them, when close he opens, spreads, his arms wide, threw them around her, she was grubbed up in an overly friendly bear-hug, — catching her off guard.

"Nice to see you again Glo."

"Hi Charles, nice to be back," she muttered.

"You are looking good. Feel good too," his flirtatious tone spoke familiarity which gored him — Thomas, right in the gut.

She had to give Charles a nudging jab to the ribs to get him to release her.

After, she took steps backward turns to look at him then made the introduction. "Thomas, this is Charles he will be briefing you."

Later he discovers Charles full name was Charlie P Tool and that he has been involved with various intelligent agencies for nearly 35 years, that he had a reputation as a doer — he got things done. P Tool is how policymakers knew him, however he is known to only a very select few field operatives; Gloria was one.

The fact that Charles had made his desires for Gloria public while in his — Thomas, presence started their, their initial, relationship off on wrong footing, he was determine to size up his competitor.

Charles had held out a hand in friendly customary. He, stone faced, allows it to hang a bit long for comfort before firmly grasping it at the same time glaring tellingly into Charles' alarmed green eyes that clash was his silver-grey hair.

She took note, felt discomfort in the fact that she had once giving in to Charles' woos, places caring, calming, hand in small of his — Thomas, back the effect was thawing, the combative handshake dissolves.

Charles escorts he and Gloria down the corridor then into a gymnasium size room.

The room was dimly lit and void of any other person, there was numerous desks arranged in semi-circles each held computer keyboard & terminal, the walls were covered with large world maps, clocks with digital tickers set to time zones around the globe, and images of dead generals.

A beam of laser light projected three-dimensional image of the globe in center of a grand circular conference table. Streaming in the background, it was barely audible, was the star-spangled banner.

He had no doubt, no doubt, that this room would have been buzzing with activity on any normal day.

Gloria, he saw, disappears into an office just off to the left, he follows Charles into another office in the right rear corner of this main room. The heavy door was closed behind them and all outside interior noises vanishes. 'Sound proof,' his mind registered.

"What are you drinking?" Charles quizzed

assuming as he pours himself whisky over ice.

"Beer," accepting the offer.

Charles reaches inside a mini-frig that sits against the wall behind desk, desk that took up a lot of space, grabs hold a bottle of Stella Artois hands it to him; the first sip was flavorful.

Besides the large executive desk, the small ivory cabinet who top held brands of liquor and a wet bar sit-up, there was two faux leather guest chairs in front of the desk, a high-back faux leather executive chair where Charles was now seated, and a faux leather sofa against wall by the door, the pale green painted walls were bare.

"You had a very successful, an excellent, conclusion to your last outing. Syria, wasn't it?" Charles starts not expecting acknowledgement he — Thomas, was not expected to answer. Charles just wanted him to know he had access to, and had read, his files.

"Are you onboard," Charles asks sternly this time expecting a decisive answer.

He — Thomas, knew that this was code talk, that no farther information would be come his way, nor would he be privy to, if he said no.

It was time to accept or decline the forthcoming assignment. He took his time, thought hard, took deep breaths, and without clue as to the nature of the assignment, with confidence, certainty, said yes.

David R McCovey

VII

"Stricken essence of stewing humanity lay scorn of vengeful righteousness vengeance I must remind is of the divine"

Reluctant Warrior

Charles stood up, walks over pours whisky in two glasses hands one to him then sits in the chair next to him, both threw down the liquor in one swift motion, sit in silence momentarily before Charles returns to chair behind the large mahogany desk were he then pulls out a gold challenge coin, the Great Seal of the Homeland insignia — coat of arms, imprinted on its face, & a unfinished pyramid, in the zenith an eye in a triangle surrounded by a glory proper, and the Latin mottoes Annuit Coeptis and Novus ordo seclorum imprinted on its back, from top drawer — flips it to him.

"The president's top advisors, those at State,

feels it's time to send Geraldo Perez a loud and clear exacting message," Charles begins his brief without persiflage nor coded talk.

"Who at State did Perez piss off to make sending a message necessary?" he, with sarcasm, asks.

"I don't think it was anyone in particular at State, what I was able to gather from outside sources points to those damn Execs over at Exton Oils, they have been complaining to the Energy Secretary, insistently complaining, about Perez nationalizing that twenty-five billion dollars pipe line project that is been constructed and, when finished, will run from Cai-quetia all the way to the bottom of the southern most peninsula. Now some lobbyist, a former congressman I suspect, got someone at State all rile about oil minister Alejandro Morales, he is the one who rejected the ruling by a court to freeze twelve billion of Caiquetia govern-ment assets, claims that the court's ruling has no effect.

It was Exton who challenged the pipeline nationalization plan in court," Charles pause his brief long enough to pour another whisky, "Minister Morales," he continues, "really got those fuckers at Ex-ton wanting blood, and Energy wants action on grounds of national security but there is no way to stop Perez from nationalizing the project so those brainiacs in the VPs office feels a message should be sent, " Charles pause again to let it all sink in.

"No Shit!" he, expressing disbelief, exhales.

"Yes. Minister Morales is also president of Petroleos de Caiquetia, he is scheduled to give a speech to board members at the Hotel Inter-Continental in Olivar in four days. We need to move now, you would have to find a way to gain access to Morales, spice his food or his drink, if not, inject him. The morning of the meeting Morales will go into a comma and the Opposition Action Party, along with the former director at Petroleos de Caiquetia, Mateo Torres, will take the blame. Everything is in place to create concern in Perez about his own safety," Charles details.

He barely heard Charles last words he was reflecting, reflecting on a career in the fight against adversaries of this nation, this nation's liberty.

Reflecting on long standing policies against assassinating other world leaders, no policy however extends to those political advisers close to other world leaders, it Morales dies due complication god rest his soul.

From when first he spoke to that dorky recruiter about a career in foreign services, and was pointed forwards intelligence, he felt a sense of pride, of duty, for the chance to serve his country in a capacity that puts him on the front line out of sight of the uninformed public.

Recalling the feel of camaraderie, of pride, after overcoming the hardship, the toilsome, grueling, 59 weeks it took to complete special operations assessment qualification.

That time, that daring time, spent at Fort Brigadier training along side future Elite Warriors has been, without doubt, an experience in self-discovery he has held close. It reshaped not only his physical attributes but also his mental attunement, the journey was not an easy one.

He had then spent the next 52 weeks along side perspective Frogmen at Amphibious Base Rona, where the first 24 weeks of underwater demolition training, and the 26 weeks of intense physical and mental, malicious, indoctrination was even more rigorous before entering Clandestine Service rudiments where he was molded and refined into a special agent for the Government of these Homelands.

Here is also where he met Earl P Roscamp a no-nonsense, take charge, son-of-a-bitch who is credited for teaching him how to hide in plan sight, how to manipulate his personality, and the finer points to recruiting and handling of foreign sources.

Roscamp was that manic-depressive manifestation he would have stayed clear of under any other circumstance.

Patriotism collides with confliction due the nature of this assignment, this silliness.

"Why are we getting involved in a situation that at first glance seems to not be a threat to the nation," he wanted some other reasoning.

"All I know is that those brainiacs, those desk jockeys, in the VPs office wants a message sent. We, unfortunately, have been chosen as the messenger," Charles.

He had never in his 20+ year career needed to question the nature, the validity, of an operation, he could see the threat to country, to way of life. This was different.

"How would you like to proceed in entering the country?" Charles inquires.

"I haven't been that active of late, I need jump time,   a night jump from high altitude would help my certification, and would be the ticket," was his answer.

"As you may know Caiquetia air space is closed to military air traffic you will have to jump from a commercial, Flying Tigress. I'll make the preparations," Charles assured.

"Good, it's a go. I would like to speak with Gloria," he, feeling resolved, announces.

"I'm afraid that wouldn't be possible, she's en-route to Dallas. She has no other role in this."

This was disappointing news, he still needed answers, plus he would have like to have spent more intimate time with her.

"What's in Dallas?"

"You have a room waiting you at the Embassy Suites, you have time to refresh. I will call when it's time," Charles got up from behind desk, walks over, opens the heavy office door, walks thru the large room into the corridor to the elevator; he follows, his question went unanswered.

"A car is waiting to take you to the hotel, there you will find supplies needed, if you have need for anything else use the cell phone among the equipment it will be delivered a-s-a-p," Charles, concluding, extends a hand.

This time he wasted no time in accepting the handshake. "How long have you known Gloria?" he asks still holding onto Charles' hand.

"Oh, we are old friends," Charles, smug, answers while taking back his hand.

"Old friends? Is it more then just friends?"

"You have a car waiting. Get some rest," Charles directs then turns, walks back down the corridor, and disappears behind the door at the far end.

He— Thomas, took the elevator back up the eight floors where Colonial Seagraves was waiting to drive him.

It was a few minutes past noon when he sled into the back seat of the black SUV with its blacked-out windows. The sky, fair and blue, was free of rain clouds, the ocean scented air carried a mild breeze, and sunshine radiated high over head.

When the helicopter had landed it was in the

darkest hours, the wee hours, time had gotten away from reality, he had lost track.

He leans back, slouching, on the seat fatigue riddled the whole of foolhardy being, exhaustion pervade sleep deprived pensive inclination, reddened eyes closes without prod as the Colonial drove though the Base gates.

The ride, coasting of the SUV, on paved road help releasing some of the seizing tension congregated in lower back. He was soon asleep dreaming, dreaming of her, of her reflective light brown hypnotic eyes, her inviting full lips, curvaceous shape of her buoyant hips she loves to flaunt, too weaponize.

Suddenly, out misty greenwoods, she, levitating about the mist, was wafting, wafting elsewhere. Temper, in heat, unfurls crystalline arms to her but she drifts far in the fading distances, temper roars out, roars out — "Gloria."

"Sir, sir, we are here," Colonial Seagraves' voice snaps him awake, he wipes away drool hanging off parted lips.

"How long was I out?"

"The drive was a little over an hour long. You don't have to check in it's all taken care of, you can go straight up," the Colonial, handing him the envelope containing room key and additional instructions, briefs.

"Thank you," he, on wobbly legs, salutes.

They, wobbly legs, exists the elevator on twelfth floor walks to end of hall to suite 1203, then enters.

It is an executive suite with sitting area just as you walk in, a small kitchen off to left, a fully stocked wet bar, a small desk with high back leather chair and credenza next to sliding glass door leading out onto balcony with panoramic view of the harbor.

In separated bedroom he found king size plush bed, a reddish mahogany chest and dresser with complimentary fresh fruit tray with two bottles of mineral water sitting on top, two matching night tables, on wall was a 47" HDTV, and to his joy a Lazy Boy that enfolds to his tired elements.

He forces himself up, walks over opens the closet it was stocked with shirts and slacks and shoes all his size. Drawers of the dresser was stocked with underwear, tees, and socks. In bathroom he found it stocked with his normal toiletries. It would seems as though Charles had thought of everything, to include his favorite brand of scotch.

"Get some rest," was Charles' last words.

Exhaustion edges resolve, he strips off the musty clothes of yesterday's freshness, drops them in middle of porcelain floor of sponge painted powder blue bathroom steps thru glass door of cultured stone shower, allows for the soaking of weary nudity.

Misting vapors steaming off hot water raining

from LED shower head fog bathroom's oval mirrors.

He was beneath, submerged in, shower gel rich lather and didn't hear the phone when it rung.

Stepping out of shower he allows water to drip from refreshed gritty skin, to air dry, using a large terry -towel only to wipe fog from full length oval mirror hanging back of door. Thru tied spent eyes stares at his own reflection, although there was signs of age he was pleased. "Time's a changing," he sighs.

A complimentary full-length terry bathrobe was laid out on bed, on sleigh bed, he slips it on it was then he notices the flashing red light streaming from the hotel phone, walks over lifts receiver, dials zero for front desk.

To his surprise, at the same time his dismay, the message was from Gloria, "I did not play a role in it," was all it said, he knew its meaning.

The receptionist, while having him of the phone, welcomes his to the Embassy and to his surprise wanted to confirm his spa treatment appointment in one-half hour.

Many of hours had pass since last he slept, he was feeling the effects.

"Thank you, but you may cancel that appointment, he, not been the spa treatment type, no he would have sought the red-light district to release stress, expresses regret.

"No problems sir. Is there anything else we can

assist you with?"

"No, I think I will try getting some sleep," with that he replaces the receiver onto its slot.

Buried among the slacks and shirts hanging in closet he saw, it stuck out like a sore thumb, the OD green duffle bag. Taking it into the sitting area, where arranged are a leather love seat, two matching chairs, and a small coffee
table, he dumps the contents onto cement tile.

First things he grabs was the .40 caliber Gluck, the box a Teflon-coated hollow point, and the cell phone, took and laid these items on the night table next to bed. Next he inspected, inventoried, and tested those items of critical need before re-stuffing the bag; placing it back in closet.

Finally he decides to lie down, as soon as woozy head sunk into memory foam pillow, sleep knocks lucidity out.

She came out exuberant mist liken mystical damsel benevolent to mettlesome loins, and came, as zephyr, naked current of exotic dream, dream of exhorting desire — exhaustion fed, floating evergreen tops of Sequoias he saw her there gaping out upon steaming ponds of dawn. In thirst hunger reaches out for her, pining her, but she morphs into falling fronds.

Carting eyes flew open, listlessly room was thinly dark moonlight filter thru open drapes, flustered brain drew blanks, memory grey, unsettling, and atop wrinkled bedding nudity lay tangled in terry robe's sway. When the first ring tone came tangles knot drowsy dull pain.

Mindful hand reaches over switches on lamp atop night table where cellular phone buzz, the radio clock reads: 0730 pm, obedient fingers flips the phone open, sleep riddled voice spoke, "Hello."

The voice streaming through has become familiar. "Everything's in play. Transportation will arrive in two hours," Charles smug tone was dry, non-embellishing.

Plans, he was confident, for his entry into Caiquetia without detection, or paper trail, was all set to go.

2130 hrs sharp. The knock on door was rapid, determined, urgent. Colonial Seagraves, dressed in black turtleneck and navy blue slacks, not his duty uniform, stood a foot beyond the threshold when he answers.

"We have to be moving; Sir," Colonial Seagraves, stoic, baritone droll hit with more thrust then before; he was in mission mode.

"Come in Colonial it'll be but a minute. I have only one bag."

"Time is pressed; Sir."

"Yes, yes, I'm on it," speaking as he exist bedroom with duffle bag slung over a shoulder.

Colonial Seagraves, still standing in hall, turns and starts walking; he follows. They rode the elevator in silence.

This time Colonial Seagraves was driving a non-descript black van. Inside, impatiently waiting, was Charles and, to his shock, Carlos massive bulk was seated on the very rear seat. He took middle seat next to Charles who on their departure hands him a beige folder.

"Memorize the flight details, and in-flight mapping. You also need to remember the contact's description, name, and counter-response. You will be getting wet so prepare yourself," Charles, locked in no-nonsense demeanor, briefs.

Quizzical, yet steady, hands opens folder — as had they have done many of times —he starts reading..., the first sheet had the flight information typed out:

"Flying Tigress L-100 Hercules cargo plane, TF-1803; departing LIX runway 3 at 2245 hrs, scheduled destination: Los Gota, Lombra."

The accompanying note reads:
"This flight is scheduled to enter
Caiquetia air space at 0128 hrs
at which time air drop is made."
The next sheet had handwritten on it:

"Mission Designator= IGNORANCE"

The last sheet, also typed, contains:
Drop zone mapping—
drop zone will be three miles off shore,
he is to make it to shore no later than 0245 hrs
at grid indicated on map,
where he's to meets up with contact,
taken to safe house where
additional instructions awaits.

Contact information—
Pablo, curly black hair, dark skin,
patch on right eye.

Counter-response wording—
'Yes, but I fancy apple pie.'

Colonial Seagraves drove the van onto tarmac of a private air field not far from Elsa Air Base.

Waiting, ready for takeoff, was a lusterless black R-44 Raven II helicopter, designed to be undetected by radar, capable of reach speeds up to 135 mph, his transportation to Los Inglas International Airport, a 40 minute flight at top speed.

The pilot, a former Black Hawk pilot, flew mostly over the waters of the Pacific, skirting briefly the contours of winding coastline, and rolling hills of populated western towns. Equipped with 10-540 Lycoming tuned-induction engine, the Raven stealthily whiz pass without notice to land in secluded field near LIXs rear gates where he — Thomas, and Colonial Seagraves, jumps into waiting lusterless black Sudan that drove the final leg onto runway 3 where Flying Tigress TF-1803 had taxied, holding for takeoff clearance.

A ladder-truck set also in wait, when expecting black Sudan crosses onto the runway the ladder-truck pulls up to door of Flying Tigress TF-1803, two passengers boarded.

David R McCovey

VIII

*"often humanity capitulates
lacking in the one thing that is
difficult too adulterate, — courage!"*

Free Falling

Air traffic control clears Flying Tigress TF-1803
for takeoff, the plane sped down runway 3, its tires
lifted off tarmac at 2245 hrs, onboard were: pilot and
co-pilot, former combat fighter pilot, and aerial bomber
pilot, respectively, now both are long range contract
pilots for the Conglomerate, also onboard with him —
Thomas, was Colonial Seagraves.

"So, Colonial, how did you get mixed up in
this?" he quiz in attempt to engage with the Colonial.

"I was a Combat Controller during the war in
the far east for special operations, I guest I impressed
somebody, after the war I received transfer orders to

Joint Force Tactical Wings, then one day I found myself on a airplane with a motherfucker who wants to know to much," was the Colonial's direct stinging response.

"I guess this means we'll going to be pen pals after this," his comeback banter.

For the first time since they met he felt a connection to this man assigned to be his shadow.

"Don't hold your breath."

With that... Colonial Seagraves starts opening the shipping contain marked with the letter 'A'. He — Thomas, pulls out a MT1-X parachute, designed for very high altitudes, from container, gave it a complete inspection.

Colonial Seagraves grabs the oxygen breathing apparatus, made serviceability check. Other item where inspected, tested, for use includes: altimeter, scuba gear, night-vision goggles.

0015 hrs. Colonial Seagraves assists with the actual donning, and pre-checks of all critical gear.

"What's next for you Colonial?" he, again trying to engage with the Colonial, asks.

"I'm going to work for Disney World."

"Yeah! One would think you would be done with dangerous jobs."

"How do everything feel? Any tightness?" Colonial Seagraves, getting back to business, asks.

"No; everything feels right."

"Ok; hour-twenty to go. You should rest your

eyes, you have a long swim."

With that... they sit in silence. He dozes off —
from out prowling gloom that lay about hedonistic
dusk ample dell a blinding grow shines... from it she
came, naked... untamed lust gleams glittering hypnotic
eyes that nabs...   plum juice ink fulsome lips flashing
pleasure rich smile... just above the screening white
plump breasts rise liken conjuring concupiscence, turns
blush regaling foliage at the hint of dawn where he
wishes soon she would come.

"Forty-five minutes before target," the captain's
ringing voice ping through clinging slumber, glazed
over eyes opens to Colonial Seagraves' brawny grin,
knowing grin.

"What the hell you smiling about?" he, flushed,
demands.

"She must be a hell-of-a woman. We should
look at map, he had it already laid out, get familiar with
the terrain," the Colonial.

Studying the topographic map with the
pinpointed objectives marked in red, he, with Colonial
Seagraves looking on, uses compass to shoot azimuth
from landing zone in the Mediterranean to the point
indicating where the contact should be.

Then calculated the swell drag effect on swim
time. "Should be an easy swim with time to spare," he

concludes.

"Any questions?" Colonial Seagraves probes,

"I think I got it. Good night for a little skydive."

"You watch your six. You can always count on the unexpected.

This was an unexpected development— Colonial Seagraves showing his soft side, his nurturing side. He had to smile.

"One last thing," the Colonial reaches into his backpack brought out an envelope, hands it to him. "Your new identification; Senor Miguel Padilla."

"Miguel?" he took the id places it in waterproof bag then into top pocket of his vest.

"Ten minutes," the captain's alarming voice broke bonding moment they awkwardly shared.

Quickly he dons the remaining gear,— oxygen tank, goggles, helmet, gloves.

Colonial Seagraves had already attached safety lines to the cable running center of the cargo hold when the red light flashes on and the aft hatch begins to open, to lower.

Noise level increases dramatically, deifying, the only way to communicate over the ear popping sound was by hand-and-arm signal. Wind swirl throughout the entirety of the cargo hold as he made his way, with some difficulty, down the aft ramp.

Colonial Seagraves' eyes was locked onto his, the Colonial waited for his thumps-up before beginning count down. On extended fingers he starts, after thumps-up, the count— ten... nine... eight... seven... six... five... four... three... two... one..., then with wave of arm points to exit.

He— Thomas, ran the few remaining steps then jumps into the void, into the blackness of night.

Gusting wind, turbulence, chilling cold, was at first destabilizing of him. For a period he fail out of control, it took all the strength he could muster to maintain the hard arch to his straining back, it took all he had until finally catching air, stabilizes, and begin to ride current, floating, descending.

A quick glance at altimeter, "18,000" it reads. He had made jumps of 20,000 feet routinely this one was no different.

The bringing of arms down along his side, the bringing of legs together, and the point of head toward surface below— together, help to increase, rapidly, like a bullet, his descent. It was to him intoxicating freefalling in dead of night.

Another quick check of altimeter, he was now below 10,000 feet at 9350, he slows descent, his plan is to deploy chute at 1,200 feet, until then he would take pleasure in been one with the clouds.

Suddenly like a mystical being, an enigmatic spirit, from out recess of subliminal orb she came forth to bring light to discipline of gray matter.

Her normally divine face was that of a tormented soul, — hideous in panic frantically shouting, shouting something, something he could not make out, could not hear, could not understand; hysterically fanning blurrier and blurrier panic-stricken arms.

The image of her flickers, liken to strobes of intense lightning, in wandering mind as brilliant, as vivid, as shooting stars raging to night darkness, — a prophesy.

And he mutters; "Gloria."

A check of the altimeter, "1,200" it reads. He reaches for and pulls the ripcord — nothing happens, nothing. No feeling, nor hearing, deployment of that cloth canopy he looks for it, for the pilot chute, not seeing neither he immediately goes through checklist, malfunction checklist, mentally goes through it again and again as the ground continue to rise.

The ground was coming closer, he discords the main chute then pulls the ripcord to the backup — nothing, no sudden jerk, no sudden stop... the ground was coming closer.

A look a altimeter, "800"... "750"... "700"... the ground was rising, panic sets in, he could hear pounding of tightening thundering heart, sweat he could feel raining, draining, beneath his garment, — the ground was rising.

"350"... shouts the altimeter. His arms, without

prod, begins to wield, to swing wildly. "200"... the ground! the ground! He heard, he think he heard, his saliva filled mouth soundless cry — "Gloria."

He was falling... The terror pitted ground was rising, with it — death!

David R McCovey

IX

"And the essential thing, psychologically, is that in dreams, fantasies, and other exceptional states of mind the most far-fetched mythological motifs and symbols can appear autochthonously at anytime, often, apparently, as the result of particular influence, traditions, and excitations working on the individual, but more often without any sign of them. These "primordial images" or "archetypes" as I have called them, belong to the basic stock of the unconscious psyche and cannot be explained as personal acquisitions. Together they make up the psychic stratum which has been called the collective unconscious," Carl Gustav Jung.

Fog of Sleep...

"Thomas!" "Thomas!" the faint urgent call, the distant call, of his name from somewhere, somewhere out beyond, beyond realm of internal world out from into wakefulness.

"Thomas!" the sound of her voice, her frantic yet familiar voice pierce the province of dreams.

Slowly consciousness itself traverse the province of dreams back into the supremacy of wakefulness' sphere of reality.

A touch, insensible senses was aroused, aroused by clutching hand shaking listless shoulder. "Thomas, wake-up," the anxiety charged voice nudge groggy eyes, hazy by fog of sleep, to awake, and subdue racing, terror amped, heart that was straining under excessive blood pressure.

Psyche was again conscious but the dream from which it emerge was vivid. Kindled mind remembers it as it was a theatrical play that leaves authentic imprints.

"You were screaming, flaring your arms. I was beginning to fear I wouldn't awaken you," Jacqueline, his wife of 28 years, spoke softly.

Hazel eyes, stressed yet delightful to gaze, was searching his still foggy light-browns for answers. He had yet to speak.

"What were you dreaming about?" she, concerned, quiz.

She is truly a beautiful woman, smoothly toned Creole skin alms of Louisiana heritage, watchful mind notes.

Jacqueline and the kids had returned soon after the storm had passed to find him asleep obviously suffering a bad dream.

After several fail attempts to wakening him she feared he would experience respiratory failure, — heart attack. "What were you dreaming?" she again inquires.

He leans over, kisses her feverish cheek, she was sitting next to him on edge of bed holding his hand in hers.

"I was falling," he, privately trying to decode the anxiety suffused dream, offers.

"Falling?" she repeats.

"Yes, I couldn't stop."

"What's troubling you dear?"

There, there it is, he heard the pitter-patter of little feet, the grand kids', hurrying about. "Nothing sweetheart, everything's fine," he fibs.

She knows him, in some ways better than he knew himself, knows he was lying but she didn't press he would tell her when he's ready, — she knew.

"Come down when you're ready," with that, she left him along with his fears.

X

"Among the many puzzles of medical psychology there is one problem child, the dream. It would be an interesting, as well as difficult, task to examine the dream exclusively in its medical aspects, that is, with regard to the diagnosis and prognosis pathological conditions. The dream does in fact concern itself with both health and sickness, and since, by virtue of its source in the unconscious, it draws upon a wealth of subliminal perceptions, it can sometimes produce things that are very well worth knowing,"
Carl Gustav Jung.

Arguments of Interpretation...

Many brainy neuroscientists who study this organ of soft nervous tissue called brain agrees — in its complexity, its cognitive wonderment, lies puzzle.

Its — brain, ability to protect, to heal, without conscious awareness may explain why some dreams are so vivid while other are so fleeting.

The author will leave dream analysis to those of advanced degrees whose studies has led to personal theories — the Freudian and the Jungians.

Here the author would only pose the question: "What affect does host fears and phobias impose on encephalon?"

Understanding, grasping, meaning of dreams stunted many a neuro-experts. As a non-neurobiologist the author, a layman, view dreams as been brain's exhaust system similar to an air tank that is under regulated pressure. When pressure, inside tank, readings go beyond maximum psi the relief valve opens relieving excess pressure so the system remains operating as design.

Dreams, the author considers, allows the brain to relieve excess worry, stress, fear, upsets of day, of week, of month, of years so host, with understanding of self, self-awareness, can find healing, as Dr Nerina Ramlakhan suggests.

The author's view may not be a new way, nor an earth shattering way, of seeing brain/dream relationship but it is however a way.

The most important argument in understanding the dynamics in the relationship lies in awareness, the basic of understanding.

"And as seekers goes through this process of change enlightened gains the ability to, and is willing to, listen to their applied awareness speak thru to consciousness."

Alone, in their Bohemian fashioned bedroom,

Thomas, some 30 minutes later, still sits on edge of sweat dampened wrinkled plush Ames wood framed bed rerunning scenes stuck on dream's projector inaptly trying to find meaning, to find courage. For tomorrow approaches.

Momentary paralysis, hallucinations of top secrete missions, mysterious woman haunting anxiety riddled thoughts, dreams of falling are all thing that may, the author believes surely, be peculiars for arguments of interpretation.

In this instance, the author argue, either or all could be the results of host not coming to terms with causation of fear, — phobia.

In reality he — Thomas, is owner of a bait & tackle shop located on waterfront of murky waters of the Southern coastline in the sleepy town of Belch.

He was, however, born and reared in a, now with new owners, tiny house on Hilliard in the city of Surfside along the coastline of the Western oceanfront. He, Jacqueline, and their three grandchildren, resides now in what could be considered the affluent part of Belch.

The couple had attended the same four year University where they met, dated, and four months after her graduation marry.

In the second year of marriage she gave birth to their one and only child, a son they named after his father.

Also as a couple they enjoy community involvements, is active in several social and neighborhood group activities.

As a local business owner he is ardently concerned with the business climate in the wider town, this is why he regularly attends meetings held by the Chambers of Commerce.

He could be counted on to volunteer, to lend a hand, when the chamber host events.

The weather had indeed turned although the grounds was saturated, swampy, some streets were flooded, and debris & rubbish was thrown about, the clouds had moved to the east leaving the skies fair and cyanic, the air was left fresh yet humid — muggy at best.

When he steps out into the brightness of day, the midday sun, Jacqueline was there lounging beneath the porch awning, the yard had been cleared, with the kids help, of litter though the lawn was marshy — waterlogged.

The house had not suffered any major damage only a few discarded shingles.

He went to sit with her, she caringly took hold his hand, places it on her lap, and patiently waits for him to speak.

"I received a phone call last night," he begins.

"Yeah; from who?"

"From Wilson at the chambers. It was about the monthly meeting tomorrow, the person that was scheduled to speak on the water front development has cancelled citing scheduling conflict. Now that committee wants me to make the presentation."

"That doesn't sound fair, on such short notice," she, perturbed, express.

"I know. And as you know I have a fear of public speaking especially when it comes to presentations. I wouldn't want the some thing to happen like in college, you remember the commencement presentation; when I fainted, passed out. It was embarrassing, I was the laughing stock, and the reason why I have not spoken to a public form since."

"Honey you'll been to hard on yourself."

"No! no, I can't do it. I too going to bow-out."

****

As exemplified in the preceding fictitious presentation the author attempted to dramatize two coping strategies for dealing with anxiety — phobia, disorder: Avoidance, and Escape.

In 1947, American Psychologist, Orval Hobart Mowrer (1907 - 1982) offered his 'two-factor theory' of avoidance learning, interpreting the development and maintenance of phobias.

His theory combined the learning principles of classical and operant conditioning, it argues phobias causation as a result of a paired association between a neutral stimulus and feared stimulus.

The author, in the preceding, effort here was to dramatize primarily the coping strategy: Escape, in dealing with phobias, through the unconscious state of dreams.

Hence; The Dream Escape.

David R McCovey

A Vow to Shadow

To have failed, failed you...

you! un-attachable shadow
sitting perched mantled ridge
with feet dangling high bustling basin

listening boisterous winds sledge
mountainous chase
midst inherit haste, of human race,

have fail to bask you in sunning grace
when lying barren lakes' thorny shores
forgive bash neglect, and rambler pace,

too; un-hide from thickets' gorge
so endeavor may stand you in nova rosiness
gifted by warming sun hallow muse

ne'er again shall you linger defaced
nor cower in scuttle darkness, —

exalting diary do avow

A Voice of Awareness

"Mysteries flourish, mystique inner world"

Proem

Social anxiety could indeed, perhaps, be a positive strive by the psyche to 'self cure' as Jung, Carl Jung, Psychiatrist, regarded it a signal that demeanor of individual's character desires growth.

Personality, he argue, does not grow absolutely, but partially with some features more underdeveloped.

Then, when these undeveloped features are ready for change, host experience the pain associated with growth. However, there can be no growth, he emphasize, without it being paid for with an equal measure of struggle.

Therefore anxiety is not something host should try to get rid of by avoiding risk or taking pills.

Rather, he argue, anxiety contains a lesson, a purpose, which cannot be found elsewhere, and holds opportunity to get to know self and latent potential. Host only role then is to withdraw into the inner world and discover what host's discomfort is asking of one.

"The inner possibility of growth in a person is a dangerous thing because either you say yes to it and go ahead, or you are killed by it. There is no other choice. It is a destiny which bas to be accepted." Marie Louise Von

Franz, Swiss Psychologist (1915 – 1998).

However, if host prefer to say no to inner possibilities, or ignore phobic symptoms then the energy which wants to express itself will surely grow against one, as Jung writes, or kill one as Von Franz writes.

The author prefer host to say yes to the possibility of inner growth and accept that which lies within the 'ethos of the soul'.

"In a predisposed person if there is no adaption for conversion and still for the purpose of defense a separation of an unbearable idea from its affect is undertaken, the effect must then remain in the psychic sphere. The weakened idea remains apart from all association in consciousness, but its freed affect attaches itself to other not in themselves unbearable ideas, which on account of this 'false' connection become obsessions. This is in brief the psychological theory of the obsessions and phobias," Sigmund Freud, Austrian Neurologist (1856 – 1939)

A Voice of Awareness 3.0

Of Mind Obsolescence

"Hence to vigorously cogitate
myriad, apposite, of matters lent
evolution of said unknowns

nil circumspection, foresight,
for certainty innumerable

vacillating obstinate aesthetic augments
tethered sagacity dilution

nil aptitude, propensity, for
reconsideration

to ponder alone in pestilent regurgitation
mired in dimming brilliance
void reflective retrospect

nil primal erudition for
applied correlation... singular.

Debased! idle mind wanders amid
pretermitted effervescence
to be beleaguered by obsolescence~

into the paltry shadows flew
dying swan once ingeniously airborne"

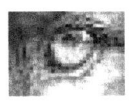

A Voice of Awareness 3.0

"In quest to obtain self-awareness seekers opt to enter a process of change, look within for answers to life adjusting questions.

For as enlightened apt to recognize, and embrace, a Voice of Awareness that is built into carnal consciousness, that by which The Creator has blessed homo sapiens with the fidelity of nous— practical intelligence.

Once ethos-of-enlightenment is allowed to guide the process of thought, a new level of awareness takes hold that comes, tranquil, with a voice that speaks through to consciousness.

Question seekers may ask, first, when speaking of a Voice of Awareness, is:

"From where does the voice come?"

Moreover, secondly: "How does it communicate with the person?"

Taking the first part, see two possible answers:

1- physiological; 2- emotional.

In exploring the possible physiological answer seekers may wonder: "Does the voice speak through conscious, or subconscious, mind?"

When looking at the second half of this question seekers may wonder: "Which of the many strains of emotions does this voice use to communicate?"

I believe, my observation, that a Voice of Awareness is subconsciously based that uses the conscious emotions of guilt, and of anger, as vehicles to communicate with the person.

The link of communication between a Voice of Awareness and the person is accomplished, intrinsically, in adverse manners. Learning to understand the language used by a Voice of Awareness can be a lifelong process.

It is my contention that all homo sapiens know when a Voice of Awareness is speaking. The goal is to learn to listen.

I believe, again, my observation, that when a Voice of Awareness speaks through the strain of guilt it causes emotional instability, physical illness, sleeplessness, and/ or mental disorders.

Emotional instability includes such frails as: Depression, Sleeplessness, Isolationism, Loneliness, Empathy.

Physical illness includes: Ulcers, Migraines, High blood pressure, Back pain.

Mental disorder includes: Phobia, Neurosis.

When a Voice of Awareness speaks through the strain of anger society, I deduct, may experience a more volatile situation which could lend itself to socially destructive behavior.

Anger is the one emotion that is perhaps the most misunderstood emotion of all. Anger is useful, I surmise, in relieving the person of stress that may manifest into other mental, emotional, or physical conditions.

Anger in itself, again I surmise, is not, and has never been, a negative emotion. Anger, like all emotions, brings about behaviors. These behaviors, I contend, is one of the ways, therein, a Voice of Awareness uses to communicate with the person.

Reasoning! The Creator's gift to homo sapiens, likely wise that a Voice of Awareness do not communicate in pleasurable ways, inevitably. Yet pleasure can be achieved by freeing the self of guilt, and controlling one's behavior when angered.

Gaining power over seekers behavior puts enlightened squarely in control of one's destiny. This freedom, itself, brings a deep internal pleasure.

And as seekers goes through this process of change enlightened gains the ability to, and is willing to, listen to their applied awareness speak thru to consciousness.

It is like an awakening of a pattern of thought that once benighted was not before aware.

Seekers can begin to put life's events, and the people that share those events, into perspectives learned from listen to a Voice of Awareness of divine self.

Making the transition from one stage of life to another seekers can only hope that a Voice of Awareness will become clearer."

DARE, O! DARE

David R McCovey

For Mother Earth

Rape of Bountiful Soil

Planet Earth~

Air at altitude, above 18,000 ft, is thin, breathing extremely difficult, yet people of the Himalayas have the upmost pleasure of living amongst earth-world most visually alluring masterpieces mother-nature incarnates.

"How much longer will it be so?" As warming clime hereafter badger winter snow...

In the remaining days, with hopes of effervescence, of tranquility, of continuation, there will be events, events that will perhaps reshape the way human socialites, interact with her bountiful soil.

Events that will be the result of how humans socialites have thus far interacted with mother earth.

Planet earth has suffered, planet earth is suffering, "Can't anyone feel her pain?"

Drenching tears raining from miaowing skies

have caused rivers' channels to overflow their erod-
ing banks,

"Can't anyone feel her pain?"

Anger filled howling winds, and torrent seas,
working in concert, has cast massive waves to destroy
places of human dwellings,

"Can't anyone feel her pain?"

Shrieking of ailing planet earth has violently
rumbled, intensely quaked, so much so new crum-
bling wounds open in blubbering bountiful skin-soil,

"Can't anyone feel her pain?"

In dire distress from the lost of the ability to
provide for all that depends on nurturing alms, she
weeps, weeps for those rare creations that has
perished, gone extinct, never to again be nourished,

"Can't anyone feel her pain?"

Menacing heat blazing from burning sunlight
that scratches blubbering bountiful skin-soil, due to
the depletion of shield designed to protect fractured

surface from exterminating ultraviolet rays, is unbearable,

"Can't anyone feel her pain?"

Robbers, industrialist, who take, and entoxicify, minerals from deep inside venerated depths causes sustaining bountiful soil to lose the ability to reproduce, is causing her sadness,

"Can't anyone feel her pain?"

She weeps in silence. In silence, amidst de void and a billion stars.

Events to change it all well happen, perhaps in future days, but will anyone, anyone, adhere?

"I absorb the waste that you heap upon me, I bear the attacks that you launch against me — why can't you feel my pain?"

All that was essential, essential to advance evolution of telluric dwellers — humanity that graze fruits of its medal; species that graze sprouts of giving loam; aquatic species that graze beneath surging oceans waves;— much was given unto all from bosom of earth's bountiful skin-soil,

i.e.- succulent vegetation that spore seeds of life.

"Can't anyone feel her pain?"

David R McCovey

The Author wishes you

wellness on your journey

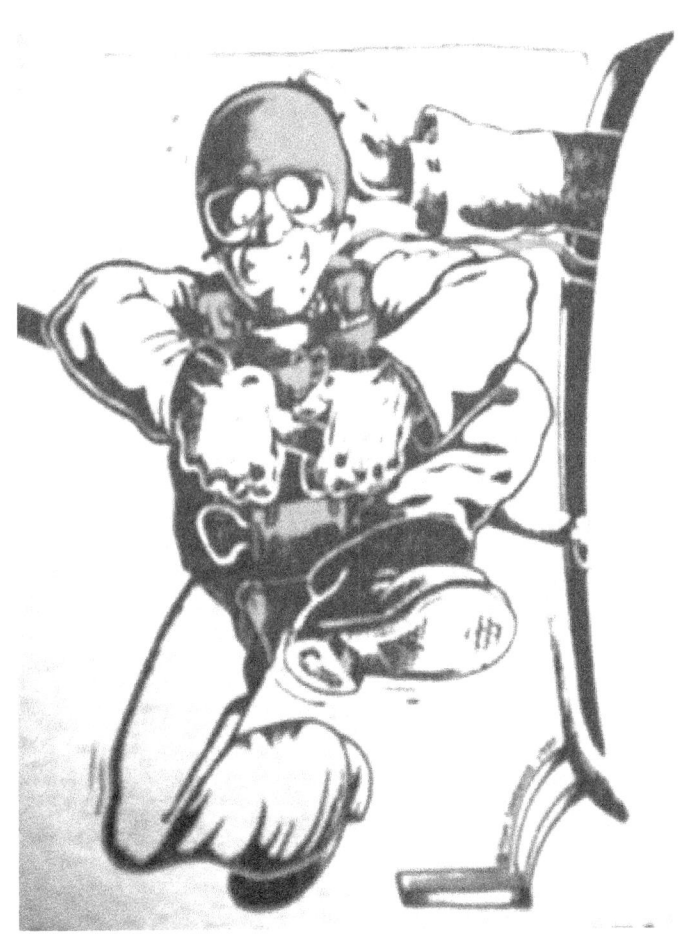

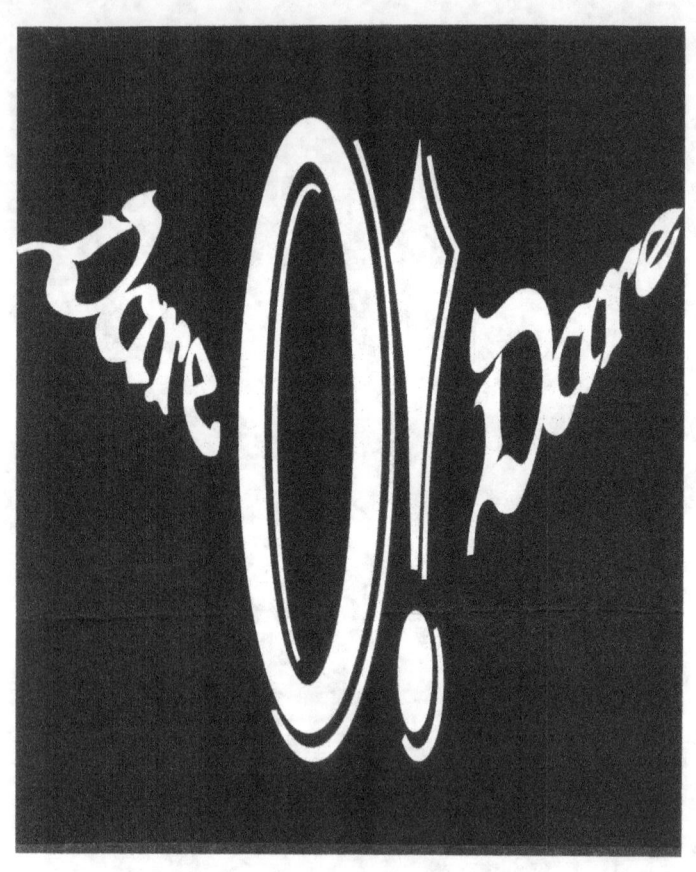